Gordon Williamson

The Ultimate Gluten-Free and Dairy-Free Cookbook: 50 Quick, Easy, and Delicious Recipes

Contents

Chapter 1

Introduction to Gluten-Free and Dairy-Free Living

Welcome to a journey of culinary exploration and vibrant, health-conscious living! In this chapter, we embark on an exciting adventure into the realms of gluten-free and dairy-free living. Whether you're taking this path for health reasons, lifestyle choices, or out of culinary curiosity, this introduction will serve as your compass, guiding you through the basics and nuances of this rewarding lifestyle.

Understanding the Basic

Let's start by demystifying the essence of gluten-free and dairy-free living. Gluten, found in wheat, barley, and rye, can be a trigger for those with gluten sensitivity or celiac disease. On the other hand, dairy-free living excludes all forms of dairy, making it suitable for those with lactose intolerance or those choosing a plant-based lifestyle. Beyond addressing specific health concerns, many individuals opt for this lifestyle to explore a diverse range of ingredients, fostering a heightened awareness of the foods they consume.

Benefits and Challenges

Adopting a gluten-free and dairy-free lifestyle isn't just about avoiding certain ingredients—it's about embracing a healthier, more mindful approach to eating. Many individuals report increased energy levels, improved digestion, and enhanced overall well-being when they transition to this lifestyle. However, like any journey, it comes with its own set of challenges. Learning to navigate food labels, finding suitable alternatives, and adapting favorite recipes are all part of the learning curve, but fear not! This cookbook is your companion through these challenges, providing delicious solutions at every turn.

Essential Ingredients

Now, let's talk about the stars of the show – the ingredients that will become your kitchen superheroes. From almond flour and coconut milk to quinoa and nutritional yeast, we'll introduce you to a palette of versatile and flavorful alternatives. These ingredients not only replace their gluten and dairy counterparts but often bring unique tastes and textures to your dishes. Get ready to discover a world of culinary possibilities that extend far beyond restrictions, opening up a realm of creativity in your kitchen.

By choosing gluten-free and dairy-free living, you are not merely changing your diet; you are embarking on a holistic lifestyle transformation. It's an exciting and rewarding journey that promises not only improved well-being but also a newfound appreciation for the diversity and abundance of delicious, nourishing foods. So, fasten your apron, sharpen those knives, and let's dive into a world of quick, easy, and delicious gluten-free and dairy-free recipes that will redefine the way you think about food. Get ready to savor the flavors of a vibrant and wholesome culinary adventure!

Chapter 2

Setting Up Your Gluten-Free and Dairy-Free Kitchen.

Welcome to the heart of your culinary sanctuary – the kitchen. In this chapter, we'll transform your kitchen into a haven for gluten-free and dairy-free cooking, ensuring that you have all the tools and ingredients you need to embark on this exciting culinary journey.

Stocking the Pantry

Let's begin by stocking your pantry with the essentials. In the world of gluten-free and dairy-free living, having a well-stocked pantry is the key to success. Start by filling your shelves with gluten-free flours like almond flour, rice flour, and tapioca flour. Dive into the world of ancient grains such as quinoa, millet, and buckwheat, which not only add variety but also pack a nutritional punch. Don't forget the dairy-free alternatives like almond milk, coconut milk, and oat milk. Keep an array of gluten-free pastas, cereals, and grains to ensure a diverse and exciting menu.

Essential Kitchen Tools

Equipping your kitchen with the right tools will make your gluten-free and dairy-free culinary adventures a breeze. Invest in a quality food processor, which can be a game-changer for making gluten-free flours and nut-based cheeses. A sturdy blender is another invaluable tool, perfect for creating creamy dairy-free sauces and smoothies. Non-stick baking sheets and parchment paper will be your allies in the world of gluten-free baking, preventing those delicious creations from sticking.

Reading Labels

Navigating the grocery store aisles can be overwhelming, especially when you're just starting your gluten-free and dairy-free journey. Take the time to familiarize yourself with reading food labels. Look out for hidden sources of gluten and dairy, and be on the lookout for terms like "wheat," "barley," "milk," and "casein." Thankfully, many brands now clearly label their products as gluten-free and dairy-free, making your shopping experience more straightforward.

As you embark on this chapter of your gluten-free and dairy-free adventure, remember that preparation is the key to success. Having a well-stocked pantry and the right tools will not only make your cooking more enjoyable but will also set you up for success in creating delicious and satisfying meals. So, roll up your sleeves, organize your pantry, and get ready to create magic in your gluten-free and dairy-free kitchen. The culinary delights awaiting you are boundless, and with the right setup, you're well on your way to becoming a master of this vibrant and health-conscious cuisine.

Chapter 3

Breakfast Delights

Welcome to the delightful realm of gluten-free and dairy-free breakfasts! In this chapter, we'll explore a variety of morning creations that not only kick start your day but also prove that living without gluten and dairy doesn't mean sacrificing flavor or indulgence.

Morning Energizers

Quinoa Breakfast Bowl with Fresh Berries

- **Ingredients:**

   - cup cooked quinoa

   - Mixed fresh berries (strawberries, blueberries, raspberries)

   - tablespoon honey or maple syrup

- Chopped nuts (almonds, walnuts) for crunch

- Dairy-free yogurt alternative

- **Instructions**:

. Combine cooked quinoa with a dollop of dairy-free yogurt.

2. Top with a generous handful of fresh berries.

3. Drizzle with honey or maple syrup for sweetness.

4. Garnish with chopped nuts for added texture.

Gluten-Free Banana Pancake

- **Ingredients**:

- 2 ripe bananas, mashed

- 2 eggs

- /2 cup gluten-free oat flour

- teaspoon baking powder

- Pinch of salt

- *Instructions:*

. In a bowl, mash bananas and mix with eggs.

2. Add oat flour, baking powder, and salt. Mix until well combined.

3. Heat a griddle or non-stick pan. Pour batter to make pancakes.

4. Cook until bubbles form, then flip and cook the other side.

Sweet and Savory Starters

Dairy-Free Spinach and Mushroom Omelet

-Ingredients:

- 3 eggs

- Handful of fresh spinach, chopped

- /2 cup mushrooms, sliced

- Salt and pepper to taste

- Dairy-free cheese alternative (optional)

- Instructions:

. Whisk eggs and season with salt and pepper.

2. In a pan, sauté mushrooms until tender, add spinach.

3. Pour whisked eggs over the veggies, cook until set.

4. Optionally, sprinkle dairy-free cheese before folding.

Chia Seed Pudding Parfait:

-Ingredients:

   - /4 cup chia seeds

   - cup almond milk

   - teaspoon vanilla extract

   - Fresh fruit (kiwi, mango, berries)

   - Gluten-free granola

- Instructions:

. Mix chia seeds, almond milk, and vanilla extract. Refrigerate overnight.

2. In the morning, layer chia pudding with fresh fruit and granola.

Whether you're craving something sweet or savory, these breakfast recipes showcase the delicious diversity that a gluten-free and dairy-free lifestyle can offer. So, rise and shine — a world of flavorful breakfasts awaits you!

Chapter 4

Appetizers and Snacks

Prepare to tantalize your taste buds with a collection of gluten-free and dairy-free appetizers and snacks. From party pleasers to on-the-go treats, this chapter ensures you never miss out on delicious bites, no matter the occasion.

Party Pleasers

Gluten-Free and Dairy-Free Spinach Artichoke Dip

 - Ingredients:

  -   cup frozen chopped spinach, thawed and drained

  - can artichoke hearts, chopped

  - cup dairy-free cream cheese

- /2 cup dairy-free mayonnaise

- cup dairy-free shredded mozzarella

- Instructions:

1 . Mix all ingredients and bake until bubbly.

2. Serve with gluten-free crackers or vegetable sticks.

Stuffed Mushrooms with Herbed Quinoa

- Ingredients:

- 2 large mushrooms, stems removed

- cup cooked quinoa

- /4 cup sundried tomatoes, chopped

- 2 tablespoons fresh parsley, chopped

- /3 cup dairy-free feta, crumbled

- Instructions:

1 . Combine quinoa, sundried tomatoes, parsley, and dairy-free feta.

2. Stuff mushrooms and bake until mushrooms are tender.

On-the-Go Snacks

Roasted Chickpeas Three Ways

-Ingredients:

- can chickpeas, drained and rinsed

- For savory: olive oil, paprika, garlic powder

- For sweet: coconut oil, cinnamon, coconut sugar

- For spicy: olive oil, cayenne pepper, cumin

- Instructions:

. Toss chickpeas in selected seasoning.

2. Roast until crispy for a savory or sweet snack.

Trail Mix Energy Bites

-Ingredients:

   - 1 cup gluten-free oats

   - /2 cup nut butter

   - /3 cup honey or maple syrup

   - /2 cup shredded coconut

   - /4 cup dairy-free chocolate chips

- Instructions:

. Mix all ingredients, then shape into bite-sized balls.

2. Refrigerate until firm.

Dive into the world of finger foods and convenient bites that are both satisfying and suitable for your gluten-free and dairy-free lifestyle. Whether you're hosting a gathering or just need a quick snack, these recipes guarantee a delightful experience for your taste buds. Get ready to impress with appetizers that prove living gluten-free and dairy-free is anything but bland!

Chapter 5

Soups and Salads

As we move through the culinary landscape of gluten-free and dairy-free living, we arrive at a chapter filled with comforting soups and vibrant salads. These recipes showcase that nourishing your body can be a delightful and flavorful experience, free from gluten and dairy.

Hearty Soup.

Lentil and Vegetable Soup

- Ingredients:

  - cup green or brown lentils, rinsed

  - onion, diced

  - 2 carrots, sliced

- 2 celery stalks, chopped

- 4 cups gluten-free vegetable broth

- can diced tomatoes

- 2 cloves garlic, minced

- teaspoon cumin

- Salt and pepper to taste

- **Instructions:**

. Sauté onion, carrots, and celery until softened.

2. Add lentils, tomatoes, garlic, cumin, broth, salt, and pepper.

3. Simmer until lentils are tender.

Creamy Butternut Squash Soup:

- **Ingredients:**

- medium butternut squash, peeled and cubed

- onion, diced

- 2 apples, peeled and chopped

- 4 cups gluten-free vegetable broth

- teaspoon cinnamon

- Salt and pepper to taste

- Instructions:

. Sauté onion until translucent, add squash and apples.

2. Pour in broth, season with cinnamon, salt, and pepper.

3. Simmer until squash is tender, then blend until smooth.

Fresh and Vibrant Salads

Quinoa and Roasted Vegetable Salad

- **Ingredients:**

  - cup cooked quinoa

  - Assorted roasted vegetables (bell peppers, zucchini, cherry tomatoes)

  - Handful of fresh basil, chopped

  - Balsamic vinaigrette dressing

  - Salt and pepper to taste

- ***Instructions:***

  1. Mix quinoa with roasted vegetables.

  2. Toss with fresh basil, drizzle with dressing, and season.

Kale and Avocado Salad with Lemon Tahini Dressing

- Ingredients:

- 4 cups kale, stems removed and chopped

- avocado, sliced

- /4 cup sunflower seeds

- Dressing: 2 tablespoons tahini, tablespoon lemon juice, clove garlic (minced), salt, and pepper

- Instructions:

. Massage kale with a bit of olive oil to soften.

2. Top with avocado slices and sunflower seeds.

3. Whisk together dressing ingredients and drizzle over the salad.

This chapter invites you to savor the richness of flavors in gluten-free and dairy-free soups and salads. From hearty lentil soups to refreshing kale salads, each recipe promises a burst of deliciousness, proving that nutritious meals can be both satisfying and scrumptious. Prepare to nourish your body and delight your palate with these wholesome creations!

Chapter 6

Main Course Marvels

Prepare to indulge in a symphony of flavors as we explore a myriad of gluten-free and dairy-free main course marvels. From one-pot wonders to globally-inspired dishes, this chapter promises to be a culinary adventure for your taste buds.

One-Pot Wonders

. Gluten-Free and Dairy-Free Chicken Curry

-Ingredients:

- .5 lbs boneless, skinless chicken thighs, cut into cubes

- onion, finely chopped

- 3 cloves garlic, minced

- can coconut milk

- 2 tablespoons gluten-free curry powder

- cup gluten-free chicken broth

- sweet potato, peeled and diced

- Salt and pepper to taste

- Instructions:

. Sauté chicken, onion, and garlic until chicken is browned.

2. Add coconut milk, curry powder, chicken broth, and sweet potato.

3. Simmer until chicken is cooked through and sweet potato is tender.

Quinoa and Black Bean Skillet

-Ingredients:

- cup cooked quinoa

- can black beans, drained and rinsed

- cup corn kernels

- red bell pepper, diced

- teaspoon cumin

- /2 teaspoon chili powder

- Juice of lime

- Fresh cilantro for garnish

- Instructions:

. Sauté bell pepper, add black beans, corn, and quinoa.

2. Season with cumin, chili powder, and lime juice.

3. Garnish with fresh cilantro before serving.

Global Flavors

Gluten-Free Pad Thai with Shrimp

- *Ingredients:*

  - 8 oz gluten-free rice noodles

  - lb shrimp, peeled and deveined

  - cup bean sprouts

  - carrot, julienned

  - 2 green onions, sliced

  - /4 cup chopped peanuts

  - Sauce: 3 tablespoons tamari, 2 tablespoons tamarind paste, tablespoon maple syrup

- *Instructions:*

  . Cook rice noodles according to package instructions.

2. Sauté shrimp, add bean sprouts, carrot, and green onions.

3. Toss with cooked noodles and sauce, garnish with chopped peanuts.

Dairy-Free Eggplant Parmesan

-Ingredients:

- 2 large eggplants, sliced

- Gluten-free breadcrumbs

- 2 cups tomato sauce

- cup dairy-free mozzarella, shredded

- Fresh basil leaves for garnish

- Instructions:

. Coat eggplant slices in gluten-free breadcrumbs and bake until golden.

2. Layer eggplant with tomato sauce and dairy-free mozzarella.

3. Bake until cheese is melted and bubbly. Garnish with fresh basil.

Whip up these gluten-free and dairy-free main course marvels to transform your dining experience. From the aromatic spices of chicken curry to the zesty tang of pad Thai, these recipes promise to satisfy your cravings for diverse and delectable meals. Get ready to embark on a global journey of flavors without compromising your dietary preferences!

Chapter 7

Sides and Accompaniments

Enhance your gluten-free and dairy-free culinary repertoire with a diverse array of sides and accompaniments. From versatile side dishes to gluten-free bread alternatives, this chapter ensures that every meal is a delightful and satisfying experience.

Versatile Side Dishes

Garlic Roasted Vegetables

- *Ingredients:*

  - Assorted vegetables (carrots, Brussels sprouts, broccoli)

  - 3 cloves garlic, minced

  - Olive oil

- Fresh thyme

- Salt and pepper to taste

- Instructions:

. Toss vegetables with minced garlic, olive oil, thyme, salt, and pepper.

2. Roast until vegetables are golden and tender.

Cauliflower Mash

- Ingredients:

- head cauliflower, chopped

- 2 cloves garlic, minced

- Dairy-free butter

- Dairy-free milk

- Salt and pepper to taste

- Instructions:

. Steam cauliflower until very tender.

2. Mash with minced garlic, dairy-free butter, and milk. Season to taste.

Quinoa and Cranberry Stuffed Acorn Squash:

- Ingredients:

  - 2 acorn squashes, halved and seeds removed

  - cup cooked quinoa

  - /2 cup dried cranberries

  - /4 cup chopped pecans

  - Maple syrup for drizzling

- Instructions:

  . Roast acorn squash until tender.

2. Mix quinoa, cranberries, and pecans. Stuff into squash halves.

3. Drizzle with maple syrup before serving.

Avocado and Tomato Salad

-Ingredients:

- 2 avocados, diced

- cup cherry tomatoes, halved

- Red onion, thinly sliced

- Fresh basil, chopped

- Balsamic vinaigrette dressing

- Instructions:

. Combine diced avocado, cherry tomatoes, red onion, and basil.

2. Drizzle with balsamic vinaigrette and toss gently.

Breads and Rolls:

Gluten-Free and Dairy-Free Dinner Rolls:

- *Ingredients:*

  - 2 cups gluten-free flour blend

  - tablespoon sugar

  - tablespoon baking powder

  - /2 teaspoon salt

  - cup dairy-free milk

  - /4 cup olive oil

- *Instructions:*

  . Preheat oven to 425°F (220°C).

  2. Mix dry ingredients, add milk and oil, stir until combined.

3. Drop spoonfuls onto a baking sheet. Bake until golden.

Rosemary and Olive Focaccia

-Ingredients:

 - 2 cups gluten-free flour

 - tablespoon sugar

 - packet dry yeast

 - teaspoon salt

 - cup warm water

 - 2 tablespoons olive oil

 - Kalamata olives and fresh rosemary for topping

- Instructions:

. Combine flour, sugar, yeast, and salt.

2. Add warm water and oil, knead until smooth.

3. Press dough into a baking pan, top with olives and rosemary.

4. Allow to rise, then bake until golden.

These versatile sides and accompaniments add flair and flavor to your gluten-free and dairy-free meals. Whether you're looking for a nutrient-packed salad or a perfect alternative to traditional dinner rolls, these recipes ensure that every bite is a celebration of delicious, wholesome goodness. Get ready to elevate your dining experience with these delightful additions!

Chapter 8

Dessert Extravaganza

Indulge your sweet tooth with a splendid array of gluten-free and dairy-free desserts that prove that a restricted diet doesn't mean compromising on decadence. From heavenly chocolate treats to fruity delights, this chapter will satisfy your cravings for sweetness without the worry of gluten or dairy.

Sweet Indulgences

Gluten-Free Chocolate Avocado Mousse:

 - *Ingredients:*

   - 2 ripe avocados

   - /2 cup cocoa powder

   - /2 cup maple syrup

- teaspoon vanilla extract

- Pinch of salt

- Instructions:

. Blend avocados until smooth.

2. Add cocoa powder, maple syrup, vanilla, and salt. Blend until creamy.

3. Chill before serving.

Almond Flour Chocolate Chip Cookies:

- Ingredients:

- 2 cups almond flour

- /2 cup coconut oil, melted

- /2 cup maple syrup

- teaspoon vanilla extract

- /2 teaspoon baking soda

- Dairy-free chocolate chips

- Instructions:

. Mix almond flour, melted coconut oil, maple syrup, vanilla, and baking soda.

2. Fold in chocolate chips. Drop spoonfuls onto a baking sheet.

3. Bake until golden around the edges.

Vegan Berry Parfait

- Ingredients:

- Mixed berries (strawberries, blueberries, raspberries)

- Dairy-free yogurt alternative

- Gluten-free granola

- Maple syrup for drizzling

- Instructions:

. Layer berries, dairy-free yogurt, and granola in a glass.

2. Repeat layers, drizzle with maple syrup.

Coconut Mango Rice Pudding:

-Ingredients:

- cup cooked white rice

- can coconut milk

- /4 cup maple syrup

- ripe mango, diced

- Toasted coconut flakes for garnish

- Instructions:

. Simmer cooked rice in coconut milk and maple syrup until creamy.

2. Top with diced mango and toasted coconut flakes.

Baking Without Limits

Gluten-Free and Dairy-Free Chocolate Cake:

- *Ingredients:*

  - 2 cups gluten-free flour blend

  - cup cocoa powder

  - /2 cups coconut sugar

  - /2 teaspoons baking powder

  - teaspoon baking soda

  - /2 cup coconut oil, melted

  - cup dairy-free milk

  - 2 teaspoons vanilla extract

- Instructions:

. Mix dry ingredients, add wet ingredients, and mix until smooth.

2. Pour into a greased cake pan. Bake until a toothpick comes out clean.

Dairy-Free Lemon Blueberry Cheesecake Bars:

- Ingredients:

- 2 cups gluten-free graham cracker crumbs

- /2 cup coconut oil, melted

- 2 cups raw cashews, soaked

- cup coconut cream

- /2 cup maple syrup

- Zest and juice of 2 lemons

- cup fresh blueberries

- *Instructions:*

. Mix graham cracker crumbs with melted coconut oil and press into a pan.

2. Blend soaked cashews, coconut cream, maple syrup, lemon zest, and juice until smooth.

3. Pour over the crust, top with blueberries, and chill until set.

Indulge in the world of gluten-free and dairy-free desserts, where each bite is a celebration of flavors and textures. From the velvety richness of chocolate avocado mousse to the fruity delight of lemon blueberry cheesecake bars, these recipes will leave you craving more. Embrace the sweetness of life without compromise!

Chapter 9

Beverages and Smoothies

Quench your thirst and revitalize your senses with a delightful assortment of gluten-free and dairy-free beverages. From energizing morning drinks to refreshing smoothies, this chapter ensures that your sips are as vibrant and satisfying as your meals.

Refreshing Drinks

Cucumber Mint Lemonade:

- *Ingredients:*

  - cucumber, sliced

  - Handful of fresh mint leaves

  - Juice of 4 lemons

  - /4 cup agave syrup or maple syrup

- 4 cups cold water

- Instructions:

. In a pitcher, combine cucumber, mint, lemon juice, and sweetener.

2. Add cold water and stir well. Refrigerate before serving.

Iced Hibiscus Tea with Berries

- Ingredients:

- 2 hibiscus tea bags

- 4 cups boiling water

- Mixed berries (strawberries, blueberries, raspberries)

- tablespoon agave syrup or honey

- Instructions:

. Steep hibiscus tea bags in boiling water. Allow to cool.

2. Add mixed berries and sweetener. Refrigerate and serve over ice.

Golden Turmeric Latte:

- Ingredients:

- cup almond milk

- teaspoon turmeric powder

- /2 teaspoon cinnamon

- tablespoon maple syrup

- Pinch of black pepper

- Instructions:

. Heat almond milk, turmeric, cinnamon, maple syrup, and black pepper.

2. Whisk until frothy and serve warm.

Watermelon Basil Cooler

- Ingredients:

- 4 cups fresh watermelon, cubed

- Handful of basil leaves

- Juice of 2 limes

- tablespoon agave syrup

- Ice cubes

- Instructions:

. Blend watermelon, basil, lime juice, and agave syrup until smooth.

2. Strain if desired, serve over ice.

Nutrient-Packed Smoothies:

Tropical Green Smoothie:

- Ingredients:

- cup kale or spinach, stems removed

- /2 cup pineapple chunks

- /2 banana

- /2 cup coconut water

- Ice cubes

- Instructions:

. Blend kale, pineapple, banana, and coconut water until smooth.

2. Add ice cubes and blend again.

Berry Bliss Smoothie Bowl:

- Ingredients:

- cup mixed berries (strawberries, blueberries, raspberries)

- /2 banana

- /2 cup dairy-free yogurt

- tablespoon chia seeds

- Granola for topping

- Instructions:

. Blend berries, banana, and dairy-free yogurt until creamy.

2. Pour into a bowl, top with chia seeds and granola.

Mango Coconut Protein Smoothie:

-Ingredients:

- cup mango chunks

- /2 cup coconut milk

- scoop dairy-free protein powder

- tablespoon almond butter

- Ice cubes

- Instructions:

. Blend mango, coconut milk, protein powder, and almond butter until smooth.

2. Add ice cubes and blend until desired consistency.

Chocolate Almond Butter Smoothie

- Ingredients:

- 2 tablespoons cocoa powder

- tablespoon almond butter

- banana

- cup almond milk

- Ice cubes

- Instructions:

. Blend cocoa powder, almond butter, banana, and almond milk until creamy.

2. Add ice cubes and blend for an extra frosty texture.

Embrace the joy of hydration with these invigorating gluten-free and dairy-free beverages. Whether you're sipping on a cooling cucumber mint lemonade or fueling up with a nutrient-packed smoothie, these recipes offer a flavorful journey for your taste buds. Cheers to vibrant sips and endless refreshment!

Chapter 10

Living the Gluten-Free and Dairy-Free Lifestyle

As you've journeyed through the diverse and delicious recipes in this cookbook, you've embraced the essence of gluten-free and dairy-free living. In this concluding chapter, we delve into the practical aspects of integrating this lifestyle into your daily routine. From dining out tips to maintaining a balanced and healthy approach, let's explore the keys to living the gluten-free and dairy-free lifestyle with joy and ease.

Dining Out Tips

Research Restaurants

Before dining out, research restaurants in your area that offer gluten-free and dairy-free options. Many establishments now provide specialized menus or are willing to accommodate dietary restrictions.

Communicate with Your Server

When at a restaurant, don't hesitate to communicate your dietary needs with the server. Ask questions about ingredients, preparation methods, and potential cross-contamination risks.

Choose Naturally Gluten-Free and Dairy-Free Cuisines

Opt for cuisines that naturally align with your dietary preferences. Many Asian, Mediterranean, and Latin American cuisines feature naturally gluten-free and dairy-free dishes.

Be Prepared with Snacks

Carry gluten-free and dairy-free snacks for times when you might not find suitable options. This ensures you always have a satisfying and safe choice on hand.

Staying Healthy and Balanced

Variety is Key:

Maintain a diverse and balanced diet by incorporating a variety of fruits, vegetables, lean proteins, and gluten-free grains. This not only ensures proper nutrition but also keeps your meals exciting.

Explore Gluten-Free and Dairy-Free Alternatives

Experiment with gluten-free and dairy-free alternatives in your cooking. From plant-based milk to nut-based cheeses, discovering these substitutes opens up a world of culinary possibilities.

Read Labels Mindfully

Develop the habit of reading food labels meticulously. Gluten and dairy can hide under various names, so being vigilant about ingredient lists is crucial for maintaining your dietary restrictions.

Listen to Your Body

Pay attention to how your body responds to different foods. If you suspect sensitivity to certain ingredients, keep a food diary to identify patterns and make informed choices.

Plan Ahead

Plan your meals and snacks ahead of time to avoid last-minute temptations or compromises. Having a well-thought-out meal plan simplifies the process of adhering to your gluten-free and dairy-free lifestyle.

Celebrate Your Journey

Embrace the positives of your gluten-free and dairy-free lifestyle. Celebrate the delicious meals you've discovered, the increased energy levels, and the overall well-being that comes with conscious and mindful eating.

Living gluten-free and dairy-free is not just a dietary choice; it's a holistic approach to wellness. By incorporating these practical tips and maintaining a positive mindset, you'll not only navigate the culinary landscape with ease but also thrive in the joyous journey of gluten-free and dairy-free living. Here's to your health, happiness, and the delectable adventures that lie ahead!